Table of Contents

Contemporary Managed Care Issues for New Physicians™

Kevin D. Cairns, MD, MPH
Anita E. Tsen, MD
Michael Witt, MD, MPH
James J. Wu, MPH

Glenn Gandelman, MD, MPH, Editor

First Edition

Published by Handbooks in Health Care Co.,
Newtown, Pennsylvania, USA

This book has been prepared and is presented as a service to the medical community. The information provided reflects the knowledge, experience, and personal opinions of Kevin D. Cairns, MD, MPH, Anita E. Tsen, MD, Michael Witt, MD, MPH, James J. Wu, MPH, and Glenn Gandelman, MD, MPH.

International Standard Book Number: 1-884065-76-7

Library of Congress Catalog Card Number: 99-66836

Acknowledgments

We would like to thank the following colleagues for their time, energy, and advice:

Annette Choolfaian, RN, MPA
Program Director
Health Services Management and Policy
New York Medical College

Cathey E. Falvo, MD, MPH
Program Director
International and General Public Health
New York Medical College

Max Garten, MS
Professor, Los Angeles Harbor College

Catherine S. Halkett, MPH
Vice President for Mission and Plan
New York Medical College

Relief Jones
Duke University School of Medicine '00

Susan A. Kline, MD
Executive Vice Dean for Academic Affairs,
Vice Provost for University Student Affairs
New York Medical College

John A. McClung, MD, FACC
Associate Professor of Clinical Medicine
New York Medical College

Richard G. McCarrick, MD
Senior Associate Dean for Undergraduate and Graduate Medical Education
New York Medical College

Gordon Moore, MD, MPH
Professor, Ambulatory Care and Prevention
Harvard Medical College

Daniel Nicoll, MD, MPH
Medical Director, Aetna U.S. Healthcare

Ralph A. O'Connell, MD
Provost and Dean of the School of Medicine
New York Medical College

Kelly A. Pun, MD
New York Medical College '99

Anthony M. Sozzo, MA, MS.Ed
Associate Dean for Student Affairs,
Director of Student Financial Planning and Student Activities
New York Medical College

Andrea N. Sullivan, MD
New York Medical College '99

The entire NYMC community

Foreword

The idea for this handbook came to us during a conversation with fellow medical students about managed health care. We were amazed at how little was known about health maintenance organizations and how they affect our training and practice. How can we be so uninformed about issues that take center stage in current political discussions and are critical to our careers?

When we searched for information on managed health care, we discovered that most of the literature did not provide the foundation required to understand contemporary issues. This book is designed to provide an unbiased explanation of managed care and its impact on medical students, residents, foreign medical graduates, government actions relating to health care, practice decisions, and many other issues.

Physicians learn plenty about technical and clinical health care; however, we learn almost nothing about the nonclinical health-care issues that are so crucial to our future. Where is the information on the variety of health-care systems, on government actions that influence medicine, and on the impact of international medical graduates? Medical school curricula include little information on these issues. Yet these factors may influence or limit choice of specialty, type of practice setting, and source of income. We cannot think of another profession whose members are so uninformed of issues relating to their salary and work environment.

Consequently, we set out to research and clarify the voluminous information on managed care. With this information, we created this handbook to inform physicians and others about health-care issues they will face throughout their training and practice. It is no longer acceptable for us to be uninformed students and doctors. We must be aware of issues that await us, and be prepared to make educated decisions about our future.

Health care in the United States is in a state of flux. Any literature written about health care today risks being outdated tomorrow. Obviously, this book presents information and makes predictions based on data as of this writing. We realize that changes will occur, and modifications will be necessary. We invite any comments you may have. We can be reached at: Handbooks in Health Care, 3 Terry Drive, Suite 201, Newtown, PA 18940.

Chapter 1

Introduction

Managed care has exerted an increasing influence on health care in the last decade. One sign of this influence is that after finishing medical school, physicians now face a health-care market much different from that of their predecessors. By understanding the fundamental philosophies of managed care, medical students and young physicians will be better prepared to make educated decisions about their future.

This handbook begins with a brief overview of basic managed care principles. The next chapter presents managed care from theoretical and historical standpoints. These theories have been significantly modified and expanded since their creation. Thus, Chapter 2 may seem elementary. It describes how managed care was originally conceived, and outlines the foundation of the systems of today. Subsequent chapters address the effect of managed care on physicians' professional lives, including medical school, residency, postresidency, and practice issues. Although this book does not cover all aspects of managed care, the fundamental principles can be applied to most managed care issues. By understanding the roles of physician substitutes, foreign medical graduates, hospitals, government, medical schools, and others in managed care, physicians can better position themselves to succeed, no matter which path the health-care market takes.

We hope that this material helps medical students and physicians learn about managed care. We also hope you become better-prepared physicians in a managed care environment.

Chapter 2

Managed Care Concepts

As of January 1997, nearly 67 million Americans were enrolled in managed care organizations (MCOs), with several million more in managed Medicare and Medicaid plans. As more patients become enrolled in MCOs, more physicians have been compelled to interact with these organizations. Health-care workers must be aware of the philosophy of managed care, the various options offered by managed care, and the differences among managed care models. An understanding of the emerging changes in health care will enable medical students and physicians to make informed decisions about residency and specialty choices, practice issues, managed care affiliations, and salary issues.

A 1993 poll conducted by the Association of American Medical Colleges (AAMC) found that most physicians were not properly trained to practice in a managed care environment. Additionally, it may take up to 18 months to retrain a resident to practice in managed health care. By learning managed care basics while still in medical school, students can be better prepared for the evolving managed care environment from the beginning of their medical education.

Definition

Managed care is a method of organizing and providing medical care to a group of individuals. In practice, the managed care concept has been adapted in a variety of different ways, resulting in a wide range of different managed care structures. Despite the differences in managed care models, one feature is common to all: MCOs attempt to coordinate and provide *cost-conscious* medical care to a group of individuals for a predetermined fee.

How did managed care begin?

As in other industries, physicians in the United States historically were paid a fee in exchange for providing a service (*fee-for-service*). *Indemnity insurance* is a form of health insurance in which a third party (eg, private insurers or the government) pays for services provided by physicians. In the indemnity system, few rules restricted the choice, timing, or frequency of visits to specialists or procedures, and this trend resulted in increasing health-care costs. Numerous individuals and organizations have turned to managed care to lower, or at least to slow down, the growth of health-care costs. MCOs have used various methods to lower health-care costs, resulting in various managed care structures.

One of the first prepaid group medical practices began at the Mayo Clinic in the late 1800s. However, the widespread use of managed care plans as distinguished from traditional indemnity insurance began with lumber companies in the Midwest and Pacific Northwest. Lumberjacks were unhappy 'passing around the hat' every time a coworker was injured on the job. Instead, the lumber companies directly employed physicians to provide comprehensive health care to all employees and to practice at a company-owned facility (this would be designated as a *staff-model HMO* by today's standards). These physicians were responsible for the health-care needs of all the patients. As employees of the lumber company, the doctors were paid a set salary regardless of the number of patients seen or how much care each patient required.

How are managed care systems similar?

Managed care systems have tried to lower costs by many different mechanisms. However, most managed care systems are similar in two ways: the use of capitation and gatekeepers. *Capitation* is the assignment of a fixed amount of money in a given period for the health care of an enrolled *member*. For example, if $100 is allotted for the health care of a particular member during a year, and that person never visits the doctor, the physician keeps the entire fee of $100. On the other hand, if the member visits the doctor frequently and incurs health-care costs of $150, the physician still receives only the agreed $100 and is not reimbursed for the remaining $50. This fee paid to the physician for the care of one patient must also encompass administrative costs, ancillary services, and other practice needs. The idea of a fixed, per-member or *capitated* payment to limit cost is a fundamental premise of many managed care formats. When managed care systems rely on prepayment or capitation—the allocation of a set amount of money for an individual's health expenses over a set period—this amount is usually expressed as a *per-member-per-month* (PMPM) fee.

The second similarity is the use of *gatekeepers* to manage the delivery of health care to plan members. Gatekeepers are usually primary care physicians (internists, pediatricians, and family practitioners), also known as generalists, who control the 'gate' to more expensive specialist services. The gatekeeper is generally the first physician seen by a member of a managed care plan. In addition to providing primary care to a member, the gatekeeper's approval is required before more expensive services are rendered. Thus, the health care delivered to a member is 'managed': someone oversees and coordinates the administration of health care. Recall that in a fee-for-service structure, a patient can go to a specialist or a hospital, often without preapproval. Additionally, in a fee-for-service system, many tests and procedures are performed and billed, regardless of their indication(s). Such unsupervised visits, procedures, and tests have been shown to unnecessarily inflate medical expenditures.

An increasing number of health-care professionals other than physicians are filling the role of gatekeeper. In some systems, nurses and physician assistants are now allowed to make major health-care decisions for patients. The use of these so-called physician substitutes, and the risks and benefits of their use, are addressed in subsequent chapters.

Managed care systems also use various mechanisms for quality control and review of the appropriateness of care provided to members, eg, *case management, utilization review,* and *quality assurance*. These are mechanisms by which the MCO can examine the cost effectiveness of care delivered to its patients.

To be certified by the National Committee for Quality Assurance (NCQA), a nonprofit organization that reviews the accreditation of managed care organizations, an MCO must have successful preventive medicine programs. Among other things, gatekeepers are encouraged to prevent disease by vaccination, prenatal care, and smoking cessation counseling. Preventive care is associated with an overall decrease in health-care costs for several reasons:

- prevention of illness
- fewer high-cost emergency room visits
- fewer overall hospitalizations and shorter lengths of stay

Managed care also emphasizes continuity of care, which helps decrease health-care costs by providing consistency of health care and retaining patients within the MCO's specialist referral system. This prevents needless and expensive repetition of tests and services.

Case Study

The Division of Diabetes Translation (DDT), a subset of the Centers for Disease Control and Prevention (CDC), fosters the expansion of preventative practices in managed care organizations (MCOs) to reduce the impact of diabetes in the United States. By designing and implementing diabetes surveillance systems between the CDC and three MCOs (The Lovelace Institutes, United Health Care, and Group Health Cooperative of Puget Sound), the collaboration can identify opportunities to improve care of diabetic patients and reduce the cost of long-term care. In particular, the collaboration is identifying the prevalence of diabetes, the prevalence indicators of more serious disease, hospitalizations, and tests and procedures performed (such as glycosylated hemoglobin levels and dilated eye examinations).

How is managed care different from other health care systems?

Third-party payers are the organizations, other than the patient or the physician, that finance the delivery of health care. For example, patients pay an insurer a monthly fee for health coverage. The insurer then pays for services whenever health care is needed. In an indemnity system, physicians often deliver the highest level of health care without regard to cost. In fact, the unlimited reimbursements may be considered an incentive for physicians to provide expensive care. In such a system, third-party payers (such as insurance companies) often pay health-care bills regardless of the appropriateness, cost of care, or benefit to the patient.

Managed care systems, on the other hand, promote cost management. Through the use of capitation and gatekeeper assessment of the appropriateness and need for medical care, *health maintenance organizations* (HMOs) and other MCOs are able to deliver health care at a lower cost than indemnity systems. Because of their potential for lower-cost health care, managed care systems have become popular with employers (Figure 1). Employers generally pay for the health care of their employees as an employment benefit, and thus choose the type of coverage.

What are the different kinds of MCOs?

Since its inception, managed care has taken many forms. As the philosophy and driving forces of managed care have changed, structures ranging from the traditional *staff-model* or *group-model HMO* and *independent practice association (IPA)*, to the more recently introduced *preferred provider organization (PPO), exclusive provider organization (EPO),* and *point-of-service (POS)* plans have been developed. These are described below.

How are managed care plans different from one another?

Managed care delivery systems are designed to control costs, but different mechanisms that they use set them apart. The chief difference among plans is the financial relationship between MCOs and *providers* (health-care professionals).

In older managed care models, such as the *staff* and *group* models, doctors are contracted by an insurer to provide care for enrollees.

In the *staff-model HMO*, exemplified by the original lumber companies and the Kaiser Foundation Health Plan in California, the insurer directly employs physicians to practice in an HMO-owned facility. The relationship between the doctor and HMO is identical to most employer-employee relationships.

The *group-model HMO* is an organization that obtains its physicians indirectly by contracting with one

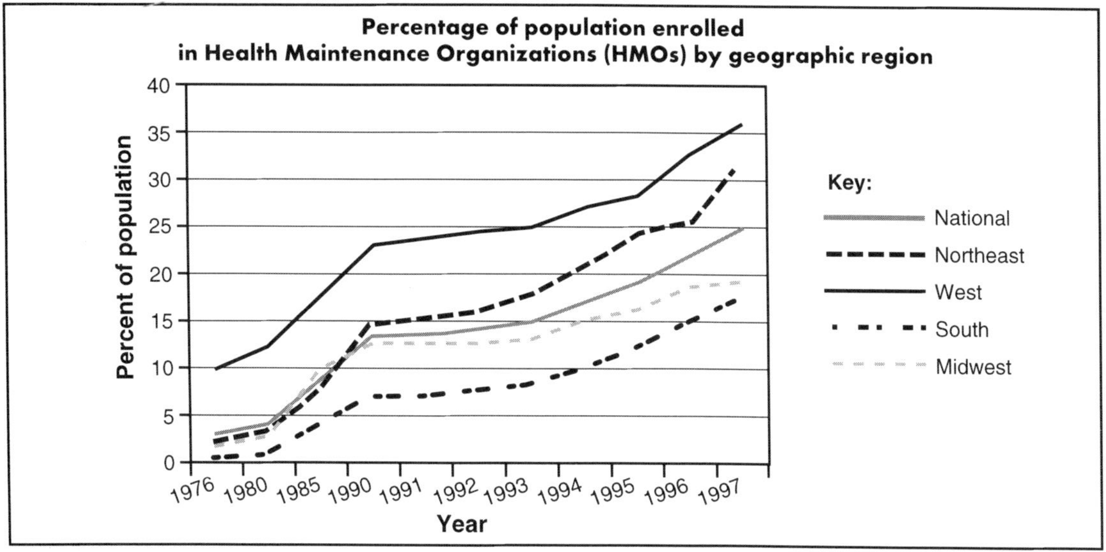

Figure 1: This graph demonstrates that a large segment of the U.S. population has been enrolled in HMOs, particularly in the 1990s. The western states have consistently had highest enrollment (U.S. Department of Health and Human Services, 1998).

multispecialty group of physicians who share resources, exemplified, for example, by the Mayo Clinic in Minnesota. The group contracts with an HMO to provide health care to its members, and distributes the amount paid by the HMO among themselves (this includes salary and practice expenses). In a group model, the group of physicians is paid a capitated amount by the HMO to provide health-care services, generally in the physicians' own offices.

As managed care became more prevalent, physicians practicing fee-for-service medicine found that many of their patients were joining managed care plans, often because employers no longer offered indemnity plans. In other words, the cheaper health care offered by MCOs was an incentive for employers (who paid for the health care) to switch employees to these plans. To continue to treat their patients, physicians began to affiliate with the MCOs in arrangements known as *independent practice associations*, or IPAs. These IPAs are groups of physicians that contract with the MCO on either a capitated or a discounted fee-for-service basis (fee-for-service at a discounted rate with the promise of high volume) to provide services to the MCOs' enrollees. One benefit to physicians in an IPA is that they can care for managed care patients and continue to care for nonenrollees. This has led to a wide popularity of IPAs with both patients and physicians.

Group, staff, and IPA plans can be further classified as *point of service* (POS), *preferred provider* (PPO), or *exclusive provider organizations* (EPO). In a point-of-service plan (POS), the third-party payer provides a list of contracted physicians available to the member, who must choose from this list. The physicians may be in a group, staff, or IPA organization. If the member uses services from one of the contracted providers, the costs are entirely covered (a small additional fixed amount, or *co-payment*, may be required from the patient for each office visit). However, if the member wants to use a physician not on the list (a noncontracted provider), the member is not reimbursed or is reimbursed for only a fraction of the total costs. The member is then responsible for paying what the insurer does not cover. Thus, enrollees can see providers not contracted by the plan, but generally at a substantial out-of-pocket cost.

The newer managed care forms are the *exclusive provider organization* (EPO) and the *preferred provider organization* (PPO). In both, groups of patients prepay physicians directly for their care. In this way, the insurer, or middleman, is eliminated, and providers are directly accountable to patients. If a member's health expenses exceed the prepayments, the providers must absorb the excess costs (capitation). The difference between the two is that in the EPO, patients can see only physicians contracted with the plan (visits to noncontracted physicians are not reimbursed), whereas in the PPO, patients can see physicians outside the plan, generally at a financial penalty similar to the POS plan.

The early forms of managed care, such as the group- and staff-model HMOs, are called *closed-panel* plans because they provide health care to members only from contracted physicians. In many of the more recent forms, such as the IPA, PPO, or POS plans, members can obtain care from physicians who are not contracted by their plan, but they are then responsible for a significant fraction of the bill. These are called *open-panel* plans. Table 1 outlines the different MCOs.

How does managed care affect physician autonomy?

Physicians lose some of their autonomy under managed care. MCOs often determine and limit coverage of certain health-care services or drugs, thereby limiting physicians' treatment options. An example of such a limitation is the use of *formularies*, or lists of drugs covered

Table 1: Managed Care Organizations

	HMO	POS
Plan design	No coverage for out-of-network unless emergency	Offers combination of PPO and HMO benefits
	Primary care physician as gatekeeper for coordination of all care	Primary care physician as gatekeeper
	Specialty referrals required	Referrals required for in-network use
	Strong incentives for in-network use	Benefit incentives for in-network use
Network (size of)	Small	Medium
Physician and hospital costs to patients	Co-payments for office visits	Co-payments for in-network use. Deductible and co-insurance for out-of-network use

Adapted from *Village Health News*. The Newsletter of the Village Health Club at Saint Vincent's Hospital, New York, NY.

PPO	Indemnity (traditional)
More similar to indemnity style	Unlimited choice of providers and specialists
No primary care gatekeeper	No primary care gatekeeper
No required referrals	No required referrals
Large	No network; entirely open access
Higher co-payments, deductibles and co-insurance	Costly: patients pay up-front fee-for-service and are reimbursed after care is provided

(and therefore reimbursed) by an MCO. Additionally, under some plans physicians are direct employees of the MCO, and are given financial incentives as a reminder that resources are limited. In others, physicians must follow clinical algorithms, further limiting their independence and autonomous decision making.

Although the restrictions placed on physicians by managed care may appear to excessively limit treatment and medication choices, such restrictions are not new. Hospitals have traditionally limited the drug choices to the least expensive drugs, and most have a formulary of their own.

What is the effect of managed care on hospitals?

Hospitals, like physicians, are affected by managed care. Much like physicians, hospitals are concerned about an adequate patient base, capitation, gatekeepers, and other managed care concepts. It is worthwhile to understand the different types of hospitals before inspecting their role in a managed care environment.

For-profit hospitals, more properly called *investor-owned hospitals*, are operated as a separate corporation or as a subsidiary of a multihospital system. In either form, this type of hospital is generally governed by the interests of its shareholders, and is ultimately controlled by an elected board of directors. As a corporation, this hospital is regulated by health regulations and by state business corporate law.

Nonprofit hospitals are structured similarly to investor-owned hospitals, with one exception: they do not return a profit to shareholders. These facilities generally are governed by a board of directors consisting of community members, have administrators to physically manage daily operations, and are subject to state nonprofit corporate law. A nonprofit hospital may also be a subsidiary of a multihospital corporation, but this corporation must be not-for-profit and function for a limited purpose (charitable, scientific, educational, religious, etc). Finally, the income and assets of the corporation cannot benefit any private individual (a shareholder, for example); nonprofit hospitals can be interested in producing revenue, but this money should be reinvested in the nonprofit interests of the hospital in the forms of improved facilities, additional staff, or new services.

Government hospitals are facilities funded and managed by a government agency. The most prominent examples are Veterans Health Administration hospitals. These facilities have a specific patient base, and the government is responsible for the cost of medical care. Patients may not have any interaction with MCOs, unless they use Medicare or Medicaid (discussed later).

Hospitals, like physicians, are affected by managed care trends, and are compelled to respond. For example:

- Hospitals are contracting with multiple different MCOs to ensure an adequate patient base.
- The use of gatekeepers by MCOs decreases the inappropriate use of specialized services and hospital facilities, decreasing the number of patients admitted to a hospital.
- An increase in the number of enrollees has strengthened the MCOs' bargaining power, allowing them to dictate lower reimbursement rates for hospitals. This trend has caused health service organizations to decrease the use of resources and shorten patients' hospital stays, with a possible impact on quality of care.
- Hospitals are subject to quality assurance audits by the MCO to maintain adequate care for managed care patients. MCOs may use the results of these audits to deny reimburesments to hospitals.

In response to these trends, hospitals have begun functioning in a managed care environment by:

- creating outpatient faculty practices and clinics, thereby reducing the use of resources in the more expensive inpatient setting;

- contracting with MCOs to provide near-exclusive care to the patients enrolled in a particular MCO;
- forming physician-hospital organizations in an attempt to regain negotiation power;
- becoming specialized facilities in a few types of illnesses or surgeries to ensure a niche in the medical community.

Is managed care making health care a business?

In the past, health care focused primarily on quality of care. Physicians knew that if they provided better health care, they would attract more patients and would thus make more money, regardless of the cost of the improved health care. Skyrocketing medical care costs and the application of managed care principles have placed an emphasis on cost and profit issues. Many physicians have been forced to contract with at least one MCO, despite decreasing reimbursement for care provided, to maintain their incomes. For similar reasons, medical centers have been competing with one another for contracts to provide care for members enrolled in MCOs.

Managed care has applied broad business concepts to the practice of medicine. Arguably, the 'production' of health care has been streamlined and made more efficient. A concious effort should be made to ensure quality is not also streamlined.

How do MCOs ensure quality medical care?

MCOs are created to provide less expensive, high-quality medical care to a large group of patients. Theoretically, it is in the best interests of the MCO to ensure quality because high-quality health care attracts new customers, retains current customers, and ensures adequate treatment of a disease to lower future costs. MCOs use methods such as *case management, utilization review,* and *quality assurance* to survey the quality of care provided and identify issues that need to be addressed. Along with MCOs' interest in maintaining quality care, the government has increasingly intervened to help ensure quality.

Case management seeks to decrease costs while maximizing the quality of care provided to patients with complicated, high-cost medical conditions. The intent is to eliminate wasteful use of health-care services, resources, and facilities, while maintaining continuity of care. Case management integrates social support structures (family, church, or social service agencies) into the overall care of the patient, both during and after the hospital stay. The MCO commonly goes beyond the contractual benefits of the plan and covers items such as durable medical equipment (eg, wheelchairs) to get the patient out of the hospital and home. Perhaps the best example of successful case management is prenatal care. Effective prenatal care of a high-risk delivery requires an MCO to assess risk factors, ensure proper prenatal pharmaceuticals and nutrition, and plan for the delivery. Improving the outcome of just a few high-risk pregnancies would decrease neonatal intensive care and future medical care costs.

Utilization review is a review of past, present, and future use of resources. MCOs use various methods to decrease utilization while ensuring adequate medical care. Some examples of prospective utilization review techniques include precertification of an inpatient admission or outpatient procedure, preadmission tests several days before a procedure without hospital admission, and same-day and 'mandatory outpatient' surgeries. During the course of a hospitalization, utilization review tracks and controls the length of stay, reviews current medical care, and conducts discharge planning.

Finally, utilization review acts retrospectively through:

- *claims review:* a method of examining large claims for mistakes, such as identifying whether billed services were actually received or were inadvertently billed multiple times.

- *pattern review:* examining patterns of utilization and subsequent outcomes among multiple facilities to identify a hospital with superior outcomes, lower costs, and shorter lengths of stay for a particular procedure. An MCO may then preferentially use that facility for that procedure or use this information to negotiate reimbursement rates with a facility.

In an environment with free choice of providers and hospitals, patients would be able to choose a physician or hospital according to their own criteria for quality. In a managed care environment, the panel of providers is restricted, requiring a blind choice of providers. As a result, patients often are assigned primary care physicians only to find that they do not care for that physician, and may choose to try multiple gatekeepers. *Quality assurance* or *quality management* ensure that providers are delivering quality care. These are blanket terms for a variety of mechanisms to assess quality of care provided by an MCO. These mechanisms include:

- *structure studies:* a large group of examinations used to ensure a safe practice environment, competent providers (assessed by a process of credentialing), proper organizational structure, and effective record keeping;
- *case auditing:* a sample of cases from a particular provider is compared with a standardized algorithm to assess deviation from standards, ultimate outcome, undesirable side effects, and costs;
- *peer review:* similar to case audits, a peer physician analyzes care provided by a colleague on a particular case. Some feel this method is used to single out a 'black sheep' who is an inadequate provider in a group, and other providers may be hesitant to second-guess a colleague;
- *procedural standards:* to ensure quality, standards related to particular patients may be required by an MCO. Childhood immunizations, prenatal care, or

mammograms after a certain age may be a standard of an MCO to ensure quality care and a good outcome. Government regulation often mandates many of these preventive medicine standards;
- *outcome studies:* these studies identify what actually happens to a group of patients after administering care. The inspection of adverse events and methods for their prevention are additional benefits of outcome studies.

Analyzing service quality, member satisfaction, and patient risk factors allows for improved medical care for MCO members. However, at some point a plan's desire to save money may clash with the patient's need for good care. Generally, money is saved not by emphasizing quality but by reducing services or shifting the costs of care onto the provider and patient.

Suggested Readings

Association of American Medical Colleges: Roles for medical education in health care reform. *Acad Med* 1994;69:512-515.

Nordgren R, Hantman JA: The effect of managed care on undergraduate medical education. *JAMA* 1996;275:1053.

Shine KI: The future of academic health centers. *Physiologist* 1995;38:51-55.

Williams SJ, Torrens PR: *Introduction to Health Services*, 4th ed. Albany, NY, Delmar, 1993.

Penner MJ: *Capitation in California: A Study of Physician Organizations Managing Risk.* Chicago, Health Administration Press, 1997.

Kuttner R: Must good HMOs go bad? First of two parts: the commercialization of prepaid group health care. *N Engl J Med* 1998;338:1558-1563.

Gray BH, ed: *The New Health Care for Profit: Doctors and Hospitals in a Competitive Environment.* Washington, National Academy Press, 1983.

Wartman SA: Managed care and its effect on residency training in internal medicine. *Arch Intern Med* 1994;154:2539-2544.

Dever GE: *Improving Outcomes in Public Health Practice: Strategy and Methods*. Gaithersburg, MD, Aspen, 1997.

Kongstvedt PR: *The Managed Health Care Handbook*, 2nd ed. Gaithersburg, MD, Aspen, 1993.

U.S. Department of Health and Human Services: Health, United States, 1998

Centers for Disease Control Web site: http://www.cdc.gov/nccdphp/ddt/projs/mgdcare.htm

Chapter 3

Managed Care and Medical Schools

Medical schools and residency programs rely on teaching hospitals to educate future physicians and to generate income. In 1992, revenue generated from teaching hospitals and faculty practice constituted 32.7% of the operating budget of the average U.S. medical school. *Faculty practice* is a term that applies to clinicians affiliated with medical schools and residency programs. Revenue from faculty practice generates funds for medical schools because clinicians give part of their revenue to the medical school in exchange for faculty appointments. A 1996 report commissioned by the U.S. Department of Health and Human Services indicated that managed care's increasing pressure on academic and medical centers (AMCs) to lower costs has resulted in decreased clinical revenues. This loss of revenue from teaching hospitals and faculty practices is greatly affecting medical schools.

The financial pressure from managed care on medical schools comes from three main areas:

- The emphasis by managed care organizations (MCOs) on cost-efficient care has resulted in overall decreased hospital utilization and lower revenue.
- Sicker, costlier patients are often not enrolled in MCOs (and often have no insurance at all). Teaching hospi-

tals are often responsible for their care by default, and must absorb these costs.

- Nearly 80% of the procedures performed at teaching hospitals can be done at lower cost in the private community. Managed care, therefore, attempts to perform these treatments and procedures in outpatient settings. As a result, teaching hospitals are faced with a decrease in patient volume.
- The higher cost of health care in AMCs can be partially attributed to research, but the pressure to cut costs has created a decrease in support staff and other research resources.

These combined pressures are forcing medical schools across the country to cut costs, downsize, consolidate, and find new sources of revenue.

To compete in this environment, hospitals have merged, creating larger, more efficient health-care organizations that can provide services at lower prices. Peter A. Kelley, Executive Vice President of Operations of New York City's Beth Israel Medical Center (now affiliated with St. Luke's-Roosevelt Medical Center in a new organization called Continuum Health Partners) summarizes this trend: "Everyone says there will soon be 4 or 5 major hospital systems in New York." New York now has more than a dozen hospital systems.

Additionally, cuts in federal grant money and decreased Medicaid reimbursement to teaching hospitals are forcing many institutions to merge and cut costs. Medical schools are decreasing costs by limiting the growth of salaries of administrators and health professionals, reducing health-care personnel, and consolidating services with other medical centers. For example, a relationship exists between the medical schools at Stanford University and the University of California at San Francisco, and between New York University and Mt. Sinai Hospital. Medical schools across the country are also constantly redefining their relationships with affiliated hospitals, and many hospitals have become independent or have affiliated with other medical schools. The next decade may bring closures, mergers, or internal changes for practically every academic medical center and medical school in the United States.

Who needs 125 medical schools anyway?

In 1970, the number of physicians nationwide per 100,000 people was 151.4. By 1996, this figure had risen to 247. Studies of the physician work force over the past 15 years have concluded that the United States has an oversupply of physicians, most of whom are specialists (Figure 1). Various groups, such as the Pew Commission, have recommended closing 20% of the nation's medical schools and reducing the number of new physicians by 10%. The managed care trend is helping to alleviate this oversupply by influencing some medical schools to merge, leading the way toward reduced class sizes.

During the 1998 medical school application year, more than 41,000 students applied for admission into 16,790 spots, about 1 acceptance for every 2.5 applicants. A decrease in the number of available spots would make this ratio even more pronounced. For example, in Philadelphia, the Medical College of Pennsylvania (MCP) and Hahnemann University merged to form the MCP/Hahnemann School of Medicine (now known as the Allegheny University of the Health Sciences). With the merger of MCP and Hahnemann, the new medical class was cut from 300 to 250 students, and has since been decreased further.

The economic concept of supply and demand suggests that a decrease in physicians would result in higher prices for medical services and more profit for physicians, if other factors remain constant. With fewer practicing physicians, demand for services per physician would theoretically increase, resulting in higher health-care salaries and costs. Higher salaries may also result in an increasing demand

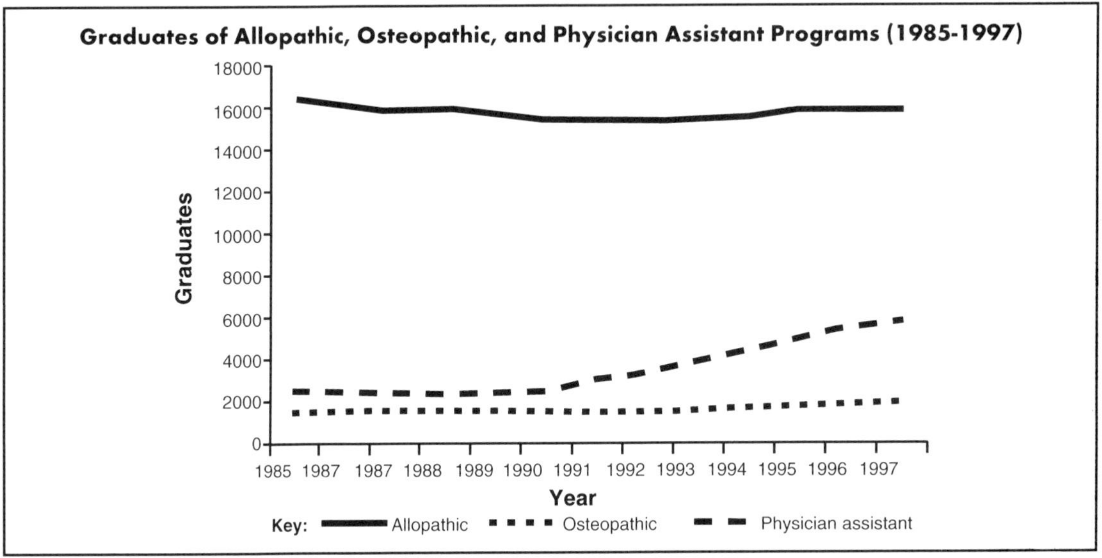

Figure 1: Note the relative stability of physician graduates with the rapid increase in the number of physician assistant graduates (United States Health Workforce Personnel Factbook, 1998).

of other health professionals, eg, physician substitutes. These could offset the decreased supply of doctors and prevent any increase in physician income. Physician substitutes are addressed below.

In 1996, the number of applications to medical schools decreased for the first time in more than 10 years, and the decrease has slowly continued through the 1999 applicant pool. Fewer applicants are balanced with decreasing class sizes, which has kept acceptance rates stable.

Who are physician substitutes?

Physician substitutes (PSs) are nonphysician health professionals, such as physician assistants (PAs) and nurse practitioners (NPs). Although the role of PSs is still restricted, they are now performing more of the tasks traditionally limited to doctors. For example, NPs can now provide anesthesia services previously performed only by anesthesiologists.

Even though physician substitutes are not trained as extensively as physicians, their services are in high demand because they are less expensive. Their salaries are a fraction of physician salaries, and many MCOs are using PSs in part-time positions that do not require a full benefits package. Thus, PSs are attractive to health-care organizations as less expensive sources of health care. Economic pressures from HMOs have contributed to a steady rise in the number of PSs in the United States.

Suggested Readings

Howard RJ: May you live in interesting times. Academic medical centers, academic societies, and the coming dominance of government and business in American medicine. *Arch Surg* 1994; 129:1123-1130.

Committee on U.S. Physician Supply: *The Nation's Physician Work-Force Options for Balancing Supply and Requirements 1996.*

PEW Health Professions Commission: *Critical Challenges: Revitalizing the Health Professions for the Twenty-First Century*. The Third Report of the Pew Health Professions Commission, 1995.

U.S. Department of Health and Human Services: *Health, United States*, 1998.

Mechanic R, Dubson A, Yu S: *The Impact of Managed Care on Clinical Research: A Preliminary Investigation* Lewin-VHI, Inc. 1996.

Chapter 4

Specialties Versus Primary Care

Primary care physicians (family practitioners, internists, and pediatricians) are the principal providers in the managed care system (Table 1). Health maintenance organizations (HMOs) rely on primary care physicians to provide most patient care, while expensive specialist services are rendered only when deemed appropriate. The managed care system can be likened to a pyramid, with primary care physicians forming the base and specialists forming the apex (Figure 1).

Primary care physicians provide most health care to the members of the plan, while expensive specialist services are used less often. Because a managed care organization (MCO) uses fewer specialists, fewer are kept on salary.

Primary care doctors are therefore used as *gatekeepers* in the managed care system. A gatekeeper controls health-care costs by monitoring patients' use of health-care services, providing appropriate cost-efficient health care, delivering preventive medicine, and coordinating comprehensive and continuous health care (Table 2).

The primary role of specialists in managed care is to serve as consultants for primary care physicians, rather than to be routine providers of ongoing services.

Table 1: Primary Care Fields

- family medicine
- internal medicine
- pediatrics

Are there too many specialists?

During the physician shortage of the 1960s and 1970s, federal funding was used to induce a growth in the supply of physicians to provide primary health care to Americans. However, this inadvertently promoted an increase in the number of specialists. Federal funding was not restricted to certain specialties; thus, the number of both primary care and specialty physicians grew. Unfortunately, the specialties attracted more new physicians, partially be-

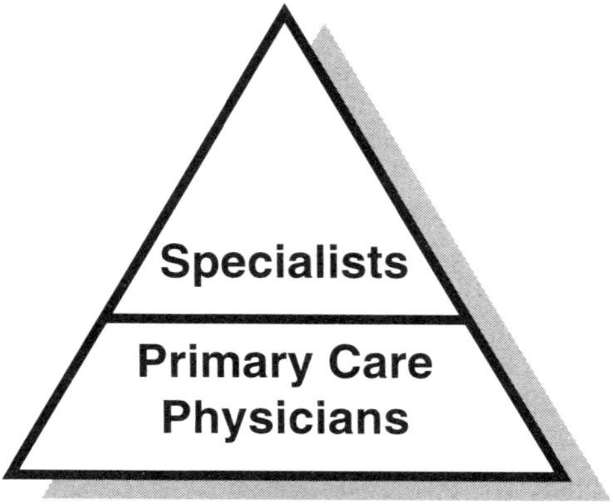

Figure 1: In managed care, primary care physicians form the base of health care.

Table 2: Roles of Gatekeepers in Managed Care

- Monitor patients' use of health-care services
- Provide cost-efficient health care
- Deliver preventive medicine
- Coordinate comprehensive and continuous care

cause of increased income potential and prestige. One study indicates that, by the end of 2000, the oversupply of specialists will reach 60%.

Supply-and-demand theory dictates that too many specialists could lead to decreased income and increased unemployment rates in many fields. Indeed, specialist salaries have been decreasing, and alarmingly high unemployment rates are evident for certain specialties. For the first time in history, American physicians are among the unemployed. Some of the highest unemployment rates for newly graduated specialist physicians reach 10% (Table 3). There is also a geographic component to the physician surplus. Many urban areas have a relative physician surplus, while some rural and lower socioeconomic regions have an inadequate number of physicians.

What has been done about the specialist/primary care physician imbalance?

In response to pressures for more primary care physicians, many medical schools are encouraging students to choose primary care fields. Special combined primary care residency programs, which combine undergraduate and graduate medical education in a shorter time, and loan forgiveness programs for primary care physicians are two common ways of encouraging medical students into primary care pathways. A common goal is for more than

Table 3: Unemployment Rates of Specialty Physicians

Specialty	Percent Without a Full-Time Position
Pathology	10.80%
Plastic Surgery	9.90%
Anesthesiology	6.50%
Pulmonary Disease	6.20%
Orthopedic Surgery	5.90%
Otolaryngology	1.50%
Geriatric Medicine	1.50%
Psychiatry	1.30%
OB/GYN	1.20%
Urology	0%

50% of graduating medical students to become primary care physicians. In 1999, 54% of graduates in the National Resident Matching Program chose primary care fields. This represents a significant increase from past years, when well over half of graduates went directly into specialist residencies. However, with only 50% of graduates entering primary care, the goal for half of the nation's physicians to be in primary care will not be achieved until 2040! This may be too slow for the rapidly changing managed care environment.

How are primary care and specialist salaries affected by managed care?

Primary care physicians have traditionally received lower salaries than specialists. Although this trend is

Table 4: The Impact of Managed Care on Specialists

- Decreased specialist salaries
- Specialists provide both primary and specialist care
- Decreased funding for specialty fellowships
- Decreased patient load
- Inadequate training of fellows

changing (primary care salaries are rising and those of specialists are falling) the lower-paid primary care physicians are still more attractive to managed care. On the other hand, specialists are experts in their fields, and often are the best and most experienced providers of specialized care. Although their fees may be higher, the services they provide are generally unavailable elsewhere. Therefore, both specialists and primary care physicians are necessary in the managed care environment: primary care physicians are important for their broad diagnostic abilities and role as gatekeepers, while specialists are valuable for their unique expertise. Although the oversupply of specialists is driving down their wages, the market should theoretically balance supply with demand for the respective specialties, and salaries should adjust to rates that reflect the market. Simply put, physicians may eventually make salaries comparable to the demand for their services.

A patient's initial contact with most managed care networks is through a primary care gatekeeper. The gatekeeper then refers patients to specialists when appropriate. In the nonmanaged care model, patients often obtain specialist care on their own, without a referral. The more expensive specialist care is often unnecessary and leads to increased health-care spending. In the past, this high spending on specialist services was enticing for new physicians, causing many to pursue better-paying specialist careers. In the managed care environment, the demand for specialists has decreased and as a result of subsequent lower reimbursements to specialists, the availability of some residencies and job opportunities has declined. The impact of managed care on specialists is outlined in Table 4.

What factors should be considered when choosing between specialties and primary care?

For a new physician, undergraduate loans combined with medical school debt can exceed $300,000, plus interest. Higher-paying specialties often are more attractive to medical students, and should be considered appropriately. For example, in 1994, primary care physicians received the lowest financial return on their educational investment, while specialists received the highest return. An important point is that this trend is mainly true for older, established physicians. Newly trained specialists may not earn as much. Although this is daunting, many physicians have entered both primary care and specialties under these financial conditions.

Lifestyle, patient base, and opportunities in a managed care environment are some of the important factors to consider in choosing an area of medicine (Table 5). A physician who desires a good living, continuity of care, and long-term patient relationships with a variety of patients may be suited for primary care. On the other hand, a physician who desires to work with fewer patients, deal with limited complex medical concerns, perform technically precise procedures, work stable hours, and be considered an expert in a focused field may be best suited for a specialty. Identifying interests, goals, and aptitudes may yield a better 'feel' for the most compatible area of medicine.

Table 5: Factors in Choosing an Area of Medicine

	Primary Care	Specialties
Patient Base	Large	Small to medium
Practice Hours	Potentially 24 hours a day	Fairly regular office hours
Variety	Large	Small, but focused
Specific Field Knowledge	Average	High
Income	High	Higher
Number of Positions	Increasing	Decreasing in many specialties
Practice Location	Anywhere	Urban, hospital-affiliated
Managed Care Opportunities	High	Average

As MCOs favor a market dominated by primary care physicians, this may be reflected in reimbursements. Primary care physicians may get more money. Lower specialist salaries may lead to a 'survival of the fittest' atmosphere, pushing some physicians out of practice. Increasing medical school costs, coupled with decreasing incomes and higher unemployment rates in some specialties, make the future appear uncertain. However, by preparing for the managed care system, physicians can work with managed care rather than against it.

Suggested Readings

Burda D: Despite big pay raises for primary-care docs, specialists are top revenue producers. *Mod Healthc* 1993;23:58.

Dunivin DL: Health professions education. The shaping of a discipline through federal funding. *Am Psychol* 1994;49:868-878.

Hurley RE, Freund DA, & Gage BJ: Gatekeeper effects on patterns of physician use. *J Fam Prac* 1991;32:167-174.

Kindig DA, Cultice JM, & Mullan F: The elusive generalist physician: Can we reach a 50% goal? *JAMA* 1993; 270:1069-1073.

Mitka M: Physician pay back up, but two-year trend still shows loss. *Am Med News* 1997;1.

Moore GT: The case of the disappearing generalist: Does it need to be solved? *Milbank Q* 1992;70:361-375.

American Association of Medical Colleges. AAMC Publications and Information Resources, October 15 , 1998 Available at: http://www.aamc.org/findinfo/start.htm. Accessed November 11, 1998

American Association of Medical Colleges. AAMC Publications and Information Resources, March 18, 1999. Available at: http://www.aamc.org/newsroom/pressrel/990318.htm.

Ward LB: Heartening signs for specialty M.D.s. *N Y Times*, Aug. 4, 1996.

Weeks WB, Wallace AE, Wallace MM, et al: A comparison of the educational costs and incomes of physicians and other professionals. *N Engl J Med* 1994;330:1280-1286.

Weiner JP: Forecasting the effects of health reform on U.S. physician workforce requirement: Evidence from HMO staffing patterns. *JAMA* 1994; 272:222-230.

Chapter 5

Managed Care and Residency Training

Graduate medical education (GME) is medical training beyond medical school (eg, internship, residency, and fellowships). It has recently been the subject of much debate because of the large amount of federal spending on GME, the physician surplus, the need for more primary care physicians, and the overabundance of specialists. In an attempt to reduce the amount of federal money spent on health care, GME has been the target of much proposed federal reform.

Who pays for GME?

GME is funded by several sources. The foremost is the federal government through Medicare and Medicaid.

Medicare pays approximately $70,000 per resident per year to residency programs in *direct* and *indirect medical education adjustment costs*. Direct costs are definable expenses incurred by hospitals; for example, resident salaries and specific administrative expenses. Indirect costs are reimbursements to teaching hospitals for the additional expense of training interns and residents; for example, costs to cover extra spending by residents because of their inexperience and tendency to 'overtreat' patients (eg, ordering unnecessary laboratory or diagnostic tests).

Because Medicaid and Medicare pay hospitals a certain amount per resident, any reduction in Medicare and Medicaid spending would decrease the amount paid to hospitals.

Additionally, faculty practice revenue indirectly subsidizes GME training. Physicians are employed by teaching hospitals to provide health care to patients, teach medical students and residents, and help fund GME by allocating a portion of their revenue back to the hospital.

Because Medicare and Medicaid cover many patients in academic medical centers, cuts in these programs would result in lower reimbursements for faculty physician services. The decreased revenue may cause physician salaries to decline. Physicians may then be less inclined to spend time teaching residents and medical students, when instead they could be seeing patients and earning more money.

Other sources of GME funding include the Department of Health and Human Services, Department of Veteran Affairs, and Department of Defense. These agencies often support training for residents at institutions they operate, such as military and veterans' hospitals.

Why is federal funding for GME a target for reduction?

First, Medicare and Medicaid reimbursements have exceeded their projected expenditure because of increased provided benefits, increased lifespan of beneficiaries, and new coverage of costlier procedures, such as dialysis and transplants, that were not originally covered. Estimates made in the mid-1990s projected that the Medicare trust fund would be depleted by 2003, but recent changes are expected to keep the fund solvent until 2015. Proposed reforms may extend that to 2027, but may also affect GME funding.

Second, the reimbursements received by hospitals from Medicare and Medicaid exceed the costs of training an extra resident, turning resident training into a profitable venture. This partially explains why the number of U.S. residency positions has steadily increased to 147% of the number of U.S. medical school graduates. A reduction in federal funding would force hospitals to become more cost-efficient and better suited to the evolving managed care environment.

Third, just as federal funding was used in the 1960s and 1970s to increase the physician work force, it is now being considered as a way of balancing the specialist and primary care provider populations. By restructuring the reimbursement method, the federal government hopes to control the number of residency positions, decrease the overall physician surplus, and adjust the ratio of primary care to specialist physicians through preferential funding of primary care residencies.

What are some of the proposed reforms to GME funding?

Several suggested reforms made by the Council on Graduate Medical Education (COGME) would serve to decrease federal health-care spending and to increase the generalist physician pool:

- Limiting first-year residency positions to 110% of the number of U.S. medical school graduates from the current 147%.
- Decreasing Medicare payment rates to specialty residency programs and increasing Medicare payment rates to primary care residency programs. This preferential funding of primary care residencies would attract medical students to generalist tracks and influence hospitals to accept more residents into these programs. This would not only increase the production of primary care physicians, but also save federal dollars by decreasing spending on longer and costlier specialist residencies.
- Including community-based residency programs into Medicare eligibility. Currently, Medicare supports resi-

dencies in hospital settings only (including their outpatient clinics). The addition of community programs and clinics, which largely focus on primary care, would produce more generalist physicians.

- Increasing funding to minority programs to increase the minority physician work force, with the goal of minority physicians returning to underserved areas to practice.

The Physicians Payment Review Commission (PPRC) has made several additional recommendations:

- Establishment of a federal agency to determine the number of first-year residencies within each specialty.
- Creation of a 'financing pool' for GME. In the financial pool, all payers for medical services would contribute to a 'pool' that would fund GME. Every residency program would need approval from a federal agency to create a new residency position; otherwise, the teaching hospital would be penalized.

Along with supporting the COGME-proposed 110% residency limit, three additional recommendations were made by the American Medical Association:

- Creation of a national planning commission to oversee the physician work force and GME funding.
- Restriction of funding to first board certifications only. Residents seeking a second board certification (eg, a subspecialty) would not have their second residency funded by the government. This should lead to a decrease in the number of physicians entering subspecialty fields.
- Creation of a GME funding pool similar to that suggested by the PPRC.

The Council on Medical Education has suggested a voucher system as an additional means of decreasing GME spending, controlling the number of residencies, and balancing the primary care/specialist ratio. Each resident would be assigned a voucher, allowing the residency program to collect federal funds for that resident's training and salary. The federal government would limit residency slots by controlling the number of available vouchers. This program would be funded by a payment pool, much like the one suggested by the PPRC. Although the specifics of such a system have not been established, the voucher system is a distinct possibility in the near future.

In the past few years, Congress has considered various pieces of legislation affecting GME, most of which call for reducing federal spending and shifting costs for GME to the private sector:

- In 1993, the Primary Care Act proposed a weighted system of allocating funds, with primary care favored over subspecialty residency programs.
- In 1995, a proposal was made to limit residency positions and reduce Medicare indirect medical education adjustment payments.
- Also in 1995, a proposal was made to create a GME trust fund, consisting of general tax revenues separate from Medicare and Medicaid payments, thereby making taxpayers directly responsible for GME.

These three proposals have not yet become law.

What has already been done to reduce GME spending?

In February 1997, the Health Care Financing Administration (HCFA) announced a federal government plan to decrease Medicare funding of GME, reduce the number of residency positions, and influence the primary care/specialty physician ratio. According to this project, $400 million will be distributed over 6 years to 41 New York hospitals, which have volunteered to decrease the number of residents they train. These funds will defray the costs incurred by training fewer residents, including the costs of employing more expensive staff (such as staff physicians, nurse practitioners, and physician assistants) to perform services previously rendered by residents. Hospitals that substantially increase their primary care residency positions will be allowed to reduce their residency positions by only 20% over the next 5 years. Hospitals retaining their ratio of primary care to specialty residencies must cut their total residency positions by 25%. If this project is successful, the government will save $300 million a year in Medicare spending, increase the number of primary care physicians, and reduce the physician oversupply. Reimbursing hospitals for training fewer residents may soon become a nationwide program.

Despite concerns that an oversupply of physicians will occur in the near future, the trend to downsize residency programs has not occurred. The overall number of residency positions offered in the 1999 National Resident Matching Program increased by 154 from 1998, to a total of 20,453. Of those, 13,707 were filled by U.S. medical school graduates.

How has managed care affected residency training?

Because managed care has a growing impact on all aspects of medicine, it may be worthwhile to ask *how much* of a role managed care plays in residency programs. The increased prevalence of managed care can affect hours of work, patient base, and type of training.

- *Hours of work*: In general, a resident's hours seem countless, especially during the first year. Managed care offers residents a slightly more stable lifestyle by having most patients' appointments scheduled during normal business hours.
- *Patient base*: Because health care (including that provided by managed care) is usually a benefit provided by employers to employees, most managed care patients are healthy and young enough to still be employed. Thus, a managed care environment may limit residents' exposure to a variety of illnesses and lessen the scope and quality of residency training. However, current and upcoming legislation may change the lim-

ited patient base. With the entry of older and indigent Medicare and Medicaid patients into the managed care market, resident physicians may be exposed to a more diverse patient base.

- *Outpatient vs. inpatient*: Managed care makes greater use of less expensive outpatient services, as opposed to more expensive inpatient care. Residents working in a managed care setting may thus be exposed to the more acute symptoms of outpatients, while having limited exposure to the chronic illnesses of inpatients. Also, patients are often discharged before test results are obtained, and residents are given the responsibility of outpatient follow-up.

Resident education in academic hospitals has emphasized inpatient rather than outpatient care. This focus has changed under managed care. Education now emphasizes primarily combinations of the following:

- outpatient care
- primary care
- preventive care/health promotion
- cost-effective care (via clinical pathways or outcome-based medicine)
- evidence-based medicine: making diagnoses entirely on presenting symptoms as opposed to performing additional tests to eliminate other possible diagnoses
- epidemiologic approach: managed care often determines treatment protocols based on community needs as a whole rather than on the individual patient
- standardized care: every patient with certain presenting symptoms receives the same health care (ie, following clinical algorithms)

How can managed care further contribute to residencies?

Historically, the task and expense of educating residents has resided mainly with academic medical centers (AMCs). However, the loss of patients to managed care and the resulting decrease in revenues has caused hardships for many AMCs. Because managed care employs physicians trained in academic medical centers, many observers feel that managed care should assume part of the financial burden of training physicians. In other words, if managed care wants to use or employ doctors trained in teaching hospitals, then it should pay for part of their education.

How would a 'managed care' residency be different from a traditional one?

An increase in the control of medical training by managed care could shift the focus of patient care. AMCs have traditionally focused on education, research, complex medical problems, and care for the poor and uninsured. Managed care focuses primarily on the efficient provision of health care while limiting the use of nonessential technology and tests. Thus, changes made by managed care could affect patient population, type of education, and clinical decision-making for residents.

One problem with the managed care approach to teaching is its potential discouragement of critical thinking. Managed care guidelines and treatment protocols often restrict physicians' decision-making by limiting the availability of diagnostic tests. Managed care organizations (MCOs) expect residents to equate a given symptom or set of symptoms with a given test or set of tests to be ordered, rather than to think critically. Other tests for less likely diagnoses are deferred unless the result of the first test is nondifferential. This standardization of medical care often saves money and creates reproducible and, hence, 'reliable' practice decisions, but may cost time in critical situations. For example, in a patient with an unusual diagnosis (a "zebra"), precious time may be spent ruling out more common but incorrect diagnoses (the "horses"). This may delay diagnosis and subsequent treatment.

What are the advantages of a managed care-sponsored residency?

- Managed care can provide residents with a stable and predictable flow of patients to learn from, as well as predetermined and consistent working hours and call schedule.
- Managed care funding of GME could be considered an investment by MCOs. Such funding ensures a constant supply of residents.
- By focusing on primary care, managed care would produce more generalists.
- Residents in managed care residencies may have greater employment opportunities within MCOs, especially in the administrative arena.

What are the problems associated with managed care funding residencies?

MCOs must provide an adequate patient base to ensure proper training for residents. This includes providing exposure to various clinical cases and opportunities to observe and manage a variety of illnesses, including conditions requiring chronic care. The prevalence of healthy patients with mostly acute illnesses in managed care programs limits resident training. Additionally, the emphasis in managed care on outpatient care results in underexposure to inpatient settings for residents in a managed care training program.

Another conflict between managed care and traditional residency training is that MCOs often prefer that their physicians use cost-saving guidelines and protocols. Yet, critical analysis and medical decision-making are integral to resident education. These are rarely used in the streamlined clinical pathways used by today's MCOs.

Managed care may solve certain problems facing medicine today, such as the scarcity of primary care physicians, the oversupply of specialists, and the immense federal spending on residencies. Several consequences of these changes can be foreseen, and some repercussions have already occurred:

- Physicians and hospitals will continue to lose autonomy. MCOs often determine which services will be offered and in what setting. For example, children with urinary tract infections routinely had voiding cystourethrograms before discharge; now, they are discharged sooner and scheduled for the test as outpatients. In addition, residents, physicians, and AMCs may be treated as employees of a 'company' (namely, the managed care entity).
- Patients will become clients, health-care centers will focus more on profit, and health-care planning could turn into health-care marketing.
- Patient load has decreased in teaching hospitals, forcing them to compete with one another and with less expensive community hospitals for managed care contracts. This competition could result in hospital closures and decreased access to health care in these communities.
- An important aspect of managed care is cost control. A residency program strongly influenced by managed care may have more interest in cost management than in educating high-quality physicians.
- Finally, the proposed reductions in residency positions may lead to fewer residents seeking work in research laboratories and fellowships. Thus, research productivity and scientific progress could slow.

Without a doubt, graduate medical education will change dramatically in the next few years, and the effects of such changes will be very interesting.

How does managed care affect clinical teaching staff?

Because patient care is more profitable than teaching, attending physicians may be less likely to volunteer their teaching time if their revenue decreases under the influence of managed care. Consequently, attending teaching and supervision may decrease. Additionally, because reimbursement is less under managed care than under the traditional fee-for-service, attending physicians must now cover more patients to earn the same amount of money, which translates into less time for each patient and, consequently, less time for teaching.

Suggested Readings

Dunivin DL: Health professions education. The shaping of a discipline through federal funding. *Am Psychol* 1994;49:868-878.

Council on Graduate Medical Education: *Improving Access to Health Care Through Physician Work-Force Reform: Direction for the Twentieth Century*. Third report of the Council on Graduate Medical Education, 1992, pp 1-70.

Hollister D Jr: Financing of graduate medical education. *Conn Med* 1995;59:629.

Howard RB: Medical education: an unwelcome guest at the health care table. *Postgrad Med* 1995;98:23-25.

Schwartz A, Ginsburg PB, LeRoy LB: Reforming graduate medical education. Summary report of the Physician Payment Review Commission. *JAMA* 1993;270:1079-1082.

Eisenberg JM: Local logic and national nonsense: financing of graduate medical education encourages expansion of residencies. *J Gen Intern Med* 1993;8:639-640.

Howard RJ: May you live in interesting times. Academic medical centers, academic societies, and the coming dominance of government and business in American medicine. *Arch Surg* 1994;129:1123-1130.

Council on Medical Education: *Report 1 Funding of Graduate Medical Education, Executive Summary*. AMA National Conference, Atlanta, October 1996.

Crimmins TJ: Starting practice in 2005? How will you get GME? *Minn Med* 1995;78:34.

Hollister D: Financing of graduate medical education. *Conn Med* 1995;59:629.

Kassirer JP: Redesigning graduate medical education—location and content. *N Engl J Med* 1996;335:507-509.

Rich EC, Wartman SA: Health care reform and funding of graduate medical education. *J Gen Intern Med* 1994;9:55-57.

Mitka M: Federal project pays N.Y. med schools to cut residency slots. *AMA Medical News* 1997;40(10):1,37.

Moran M: Match offers more residency slots–but not for IMGs. *AMA Medical News*, April 6, 1998.

Wartman SA: Managed care and its effect on residency training in internal medicine. *Arch Intern Med* 1994;154:2539-2544.

Kuttner R: Must good HMOs go bad? First of two parts: the commercialization of prepaid group health care. *N Engl J Med* 1998;338:1558-1563.

Corrigan JM, Thompson LM: Contractual arrangements between residency programs and HMOs. *J Fam Pract* 1992;35:543-547.

American Association of Medical Colleges. AAMC Publications and Information Resources, March 18, 1999. Available at: http://www.aamc.org/newsroom/pressrel/990318.htm.

Chapter 6

Foreign Medical Graduates and Residency Opportunities

Foreign medical graduates (FMGs) and their newer name, international medical graduates (IMGs), are graduates of medical schools outside of the U.S., Puerto Rico, and Canada. The two main types of IMGs are:

- U.S. citizens who went to medical school abroad
- Foreign nationals (not U.S. citizens) who graduated from foreign medical schools

Why does the U.S. allow IMGs into residency programs?

- The threat of a physician shortage in the 1960s and 1970s led the government to loosen immigration restrictions for physicians who wanted to enter the U.S.
- Allowing an IMG to train in the United States benefits the international graduate, who receives an advanced medical education while providing medical services at U.S. teaching hospitals.
- Upon return to their native countries, IMGs bring with them the best of U.S. medical training. Their skills and

knowledge can then benefit patients in their native countries.

How do IMGs affect U.S. medical graduates?

In 1993, about 25,000 residency slots were available. This number represents 147% of the number of U.S. medical school graduates, virtually guaranteeing a residency position to every graduating U.S. medical student. However, the perceived physician surplus has made this percentage a target for reduction by the government, the American Medical Association, and others. The proposed limit on first-year residency positions to 110% of U.S. medical school graduates could create some difficulty for U.S. medical graduates.

IMGs apply for the same residency spots, making the field more competitive for U.S. medical graduates in obtaining their desired residency. However, U.S. teaching hospitals have been known to prefer U.S. medical graduates to IMGs. Although the 110% limit may not hinder U.S. medical graduates from obtaining a residency position, decreased positions in desirable residencies will drive U.S. medical graduates into the less desirable residencies.

How will IMGs be affected by the 110% limit?

Although U.S. medical graduates obtain a residency position, IMGs will find it difficult to obtain residency positions. IMGs who are U.S. citizens (and often have better English proficiency) are preferred over IMGs not from the United States. However, regardless of citizenship, many residency programs may not accept IMGs because of biases and difficulties in evaluating their credentials. Thus, IMGs will bear the brunt of the reductions imposed by past reductions and the proposed residency position limit. In 1998, the number of IMGs matching into U.S. residency programs fell by 3% to 7,957, the first such decrease in 6 years (Figure 1).

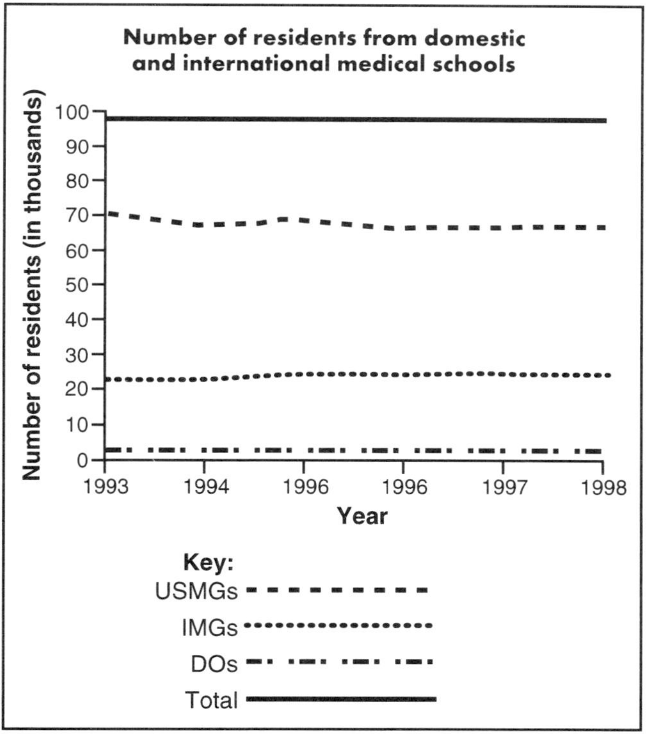

Figure 1: Despite much debate about limiting the total number of physicians and the number of international graduates, the total number of residents in training is fairly constant and the number of IMGs has slowly increased (Presented from data from Miller RS, Dunn MR, Richter T: Graduate medical education, 1998-1999. *JAMA* 1999: 282:885-850).

Are there problems associated with decreasing the number of IMGs?

IMGs often train in residency programs least favored by U.S. medical graduates, such as those in less popular specialties or geographic locations. Any limitations on the number of IMGs allowed to enter the United States could leave these residencies and hospitals understaffed. Because many of the undesirable residencies are in underserved areas, the result will be a devastating shortage of physicians in certain communities. Hospitals in some inner cities have depended heavily on IMGs to fill their residency positions. Limiting the number of IMGs may limit these hospitals' ability to hire a sufficient number of residents to provide patient care.

Does the U.S. still need IMGs?

During the physician shortage of the 1960s and 1970s, the United States government sought to increase the supply of generalist physicians and to populate medically underserved areas with more doctors. More medical schools, increased class sizes, and immigration of more IMGs all contributed to increasing the number of physicians. Although the policies were intended to solve the physician shortage of the 1960s and 1970s, they created a new problem in the 1980s and 1990s. IMGs are needed to fill residency positions in underserved areas; however, recent studies show that they do not remain in these areas after their residencies. IMGs tend to settle in the same areas as U.S. medical graduates, namely, urban communities with adequate physician populations. IMGs appear to choose residencies in primary care, but few stay in primary care. Many proceed to specialize, even more so than their U.S. medical graduate counterparts.

IMGs are admitted with the provision that they return to their native country when their training is completed, but many do not return. Most IMGs who enter the United States ultimately stay here, thus contributing to the physician surplus and the generalist/specialist imbalance. The nearly 5,000 IMGs who enter the United States every year represent the equivalent of 50 international medical school graduating classes. Is it fair to allow so many bright students to leave their homelands with no intention of returning? Some consider this 'brain-drain' an unfair immigration policy.

With the current oversupply of physicians, legislation to limit the physician population is inevitable. By decreasing the number of IMGs, the government can quickly and significantly curb the U.S. physician population.

Suggested Readings

American College of Physicians: The physician workforce and financing of graduate medical education. *Ann Intern Med* 1998;128:142-148.

Moran M: Match offers more residency slots—but not for IMGs. *AMA Medical News*, April 6, 1998.

Mullan F, Politzer RM, Davis CH: Medical migration and the physician workforce. International medical graduates and American medicine. *JAMA* 1995;273:1521-1527.

Chapter 7

Postresidency Training

Postresidency is additional training in a specialized field of medicine beyond the residency years. Typically, it takes the form of a fellowship that lasts 1 to 5 years. A fellowship can also be considered a transitional phase between residency and a possible career involving research, teaching, or other health-related areas. Almost half of all graduates from MD programs enter internal medicine or pediatric residencies; 60% of internal medicine residents and 40% of pediatric residents enter subspecialty fellowships. Whether fellowships produce better-skilled physicians is arguable; however, postresidency training undoubtedly provides physicians with an opportunity to incorporate in-depth knowledge and research into their clinical training. Table 1 lists some specialties that offer fellowships.

In the past, fellowships often led to higher income, but entering a specialty now invites a risk of unemployment in the managed care marketplace (see Chapter 4). Very few statistics are available regarding physician unemployment and underemployment. Traditional indicators for employment rates do not now support a physician excess, but changes such as increased demand for primary care residency positions and decreased demand for some specialty residencies,

Table 1: Examples of Specialty Areas Offering Fellowships

- Anesthesiology
- Cardiology
- Clinical pharmacology
- Dermatology and training
- Emergency medicine
- Geriatric psychiatry
- Health services research and development
- Obstetrics
- Ophthalmology
- Otolaryngology
- Pediatrics
- Psychiatry research
- Spinal cord injuries
- Substance abuse
- Surgery

For more information, contact the National Institutes of Health (NIH).

increased demand for physicians to retrain into primary care, and change in relative incomes for physicians, could be summarized as a shift from favor of specialist positions. Wennberg and colleagues have speculated that more than half of all specialists would be unemployed if the influence of managed care organizations (MCOs) had been present throughout the country.

Another pathway of postresidency training is medical research, either in the basic or the clinical sciences, which is necessary to expand the knowledge for treating disease. With the pursuit of lower costs by MCOs, funding for research on drugs and procedures deemed experimental is likely to decrease. Basic science research will be most affected by managed care because of its low profit potential. Clinical research, on the other hand, is often funded by private organizations such as drug manufacturers, making it more resistant to the

Table 2: Nonclinical Careers for Physicians

- Basic science research
- Health-care administration
- Medical school administration
- Health-care law/policy
- Public health

impact of managed care. With these changes in research funding, many residents may choose not to pursue training in basic science research.

Administration is another attractive option for physicians after their residencies. Managed care, as an industry, has a high demand for physicians as medical directors, upper-level managers, consultants, and appeals reviewers. Additionally, physicians may opt to involve themselves in hospital or public health program management, or in medical school administration.

Finally, some physicians may feel unprepared for the managed care environment, or may just want to pursue a different facet of medicine, and return to school. These physicians may return to school for a professional law degree, a Master of Business Administration (MBA), a Master of Public Health (MPH), or a Master of Health Administration (MHA). Some graduate schools have even designed programs toward these degrees especially for physicians. Table 2 lists some nonclinical career options for physicians.

What are the benefits of postresidency training?

- Postresidency training is required for most subspecialties and for entry into many academic and research positions.

- The investigative element of some postresidency programs may be appealing to those interested in research.
- Physicians in postresidency training have opportunities to work with some of the most knowledgeable physicians in their field, and will be exposed to new advances in these specialties.
- The mere possession of a fellowship certificate may lead to higher income opportunities in the specialty area, especially because this gives future specialists time to accumulate more patients for their patient base.

What are the disadvantages of postresidency training?

- Fellowship salaries are comparable to those of regular residency programs; some fellowships actually pay less. With a large debt incurred during medical school and the extended training time, most residents choose a higher-salary clinical position upon completion of residency training.
- Postresidency training may lack broad-based training. The clinical and laboratory experience for these physicians tends to be narrow and quite focused.
- Some fellowship programs are not accredited, and some are poorly structured and undersupervised.
- Admission to many fellowships is highly competitive, and positions are difficult to obtain.
- A postresidency fellowship program could close in the middle of training because of lack of funding.
- Employment may be difficult to obtain because of decreased use of specialists by managed care.

Do fellowships make sense in a world of managed care?

Managed care limits access to and use of expensive specialist care. The resulting decreased demand for specialist physicians has led to lower salaries. With greater need for primary care services, specialist physicians may find themselves providing more primary rather than specialist care. Additionally, the oversupply of specialists makes the use of federal funds for the additional years of training appear wasteful; thus, this has become a target for legislative reform. A large number of specialists would also decrease each individual physician's patient load, leading to insufficient exposure to challenging cases. Thus, specialist physicians would find it difficult to remain current and proficient in their specialty. Finally, in-hospital stays are decreasing under managed care. Because most postresidency training programs depend on the high patient volume of academic medical centers, those most influenced by managed care may not obtain sufficient exposure for adequate training.

Conversely, there will always be a need for specialty physicians. There is a niche for specialists that needs to be filled to provide adequate patient care.

Suggested Readings

Littlefield JW: The need to promote careers that combine research and clinical care. *J Med Educ* 1986;61:785-789.

Rivo ML, Satcher D: Improving access to health care through physician workforce reform. Directions for the 21st century. *JAMA* 1993;270:1074-1078.

Welner AH: The future of post-residency fellowship education. *Mil Med* 1993;158:236-248.

Weiner AH: Factors influencing the pursuit of careers in academic medicine: a survey of MD-Ph.D. residents in dermatology programs in the United States. *J Invest Dermatol* 1992;98:125-127.

American College of Physicians: The physician workforce and financing of graduate medical education. *Ann Intern Med* 1998;128:142-148.

Politzer RM, Gamliel SR, Cultice JM, et al: Matching physician supply and requirements: testing policy recommendations. *Inquiry* 1996;33:181-194.

Schroeder SA: Training an appropriate mix of physicians to meet the nation's needs. *Acad Med* 1993;68:118-122.

Goodman L: Managed care's role in shaping the physician market. *JAMA* 1997;277:72.

Schwartz AD: Will competition change the physician workforce? Early signals from the market. *Acad Med* 1996;71:15-22.

Wennberg JE, Goodman DC, Nease RF, et al: Finding equilibrium in U.S. physician supply. *Health Aff* 1993;12:89-103.

Chapter 8

Managed Care and Practice Issues

Among the many changes in medicine under managed care, recent reports have shown that physicians' salaries are obviously affected. The specialist fields are showing the greatest decreases in salary. This is largely because managed care plans are now offering primary care physicians substantially higher starting salaries compared to a few years ago, while specialist salaries have actually declined. Furthermore, specialist reimbursement fee scales have been progressively reduced. Additionally, managed care has affected everything from physicians' autonomy (see Chapter 2) to patient volume (Figure 1).

Who do managed care plans hire?

Managed care plans have begun to measure physician performance in several ways. Most plans have developed clinical pathways or outcome management as ways to monitor and grade physicians' performance. Clinical pathways are predetermined treatment guidelines used by physicians in managed care organizations (MCOs). Doctors who use a disproportionate share of services (especially those outside a given clinical pathway) or whose patients have longer average length of stays for a given period are awarded lower grades, and may not be offered a new con-

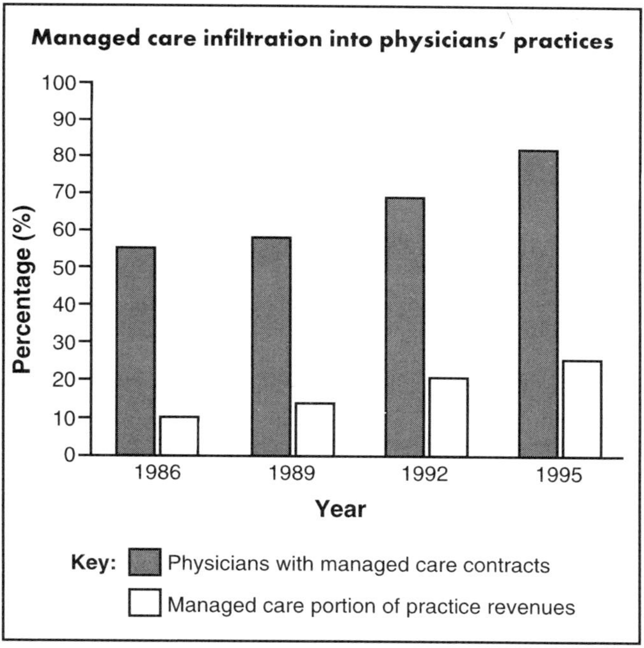

Figure 1: Between 1986 and 1995, the number of physicians with at least one managed care contract grew nearly 28%, and the amount of managed care revenues more than doubled (Presented from data from Mitka M: Doctors opt for employment, larger groups. *AMNews* January 20, 1997).

tract with the MCO. This process is known as de-selection. This has been called *economic credentialing* and has become controversial because it limits physician autonomy in clinical decision-making.

How does managed care affect individual physicians?

In addition to loss of autonomy, physicians are fearful of the new and unfamiliar health-care system under managed care. Physicians often associate managed care with answering to a less-educated nonclinician. To soften the blow from managed care, many physicians have turned to physician-driven independent practice associations (IPAs), the organizations most similar to traditional fee-for-service health-care delivery. By joining an IPA, physicians continue to practice in a setting similar to their previous fee-for-service, but are better able to compete in the marketplace with other MCOs. In 1994, IPAs were the most common type of HMO, representing 65% of all operating HMOs and accounting for 36% of enrollment in the 25 largest HMOs.

Although MCOs usually do not directly enforce limitations on how physicians spend time with patients, they do, however, often require providers to see a large number of patients in a given amount of time, thereby indirectly limiting the time spent on each patient. These time limits are designed to boost productivity, and are often referred to as *productivity guidelines*. MCOs believe these guidelines streamline care, but most physicians dislike being told how much time they are allowed to spend with a patient.

Can physicians join together to compete with HMOs?

In the past, economic alliances among physicians were limited by antitrust guidelines issued by the Department of Justice and the Federal Trade Commission (FTC). In the early 1990s, a federal court convicted three dentists of price fixing in *United States v Alston et al*. This case sent a clear message to physicians that forming economic unions was illegal because they were considered harmful to competition. In contrast, the Department of Justice and the FTC strongly advocated allowing HMOs to set reimbursement dates for the physicians working under their plans. Thus, independent physicians were strongly discouraged from forming their own networks, but were encouraged to join an HMO. This greatly hampered the ability of solo and other non-HMO physicians to compete with the organized managed care system. Additionally, physicians who are self-employed or in independent practice are not eligible to join unions. Although physicians have argued that HMOs have effectively made them employees by controlling working conditions, medical decisions, and incomes, the National Labor Relations Board has not yet agreed. However, in the fall of 1996, new guidelines were issued that recognize that physician groups (such as exclusive provider organizations [EPOs] and preferred provider organizations [PPOs]) actually represent greater market competition, and are no longer considered in violation of antitrust laws by the Department of Justice and the FTC. Physicians have thus gained greater legal flexibility to collaborate, negotiate prices, and compete with MCOs.

In mid-1999, the AMA estimated about 20,000 physicians nationwide belonged to such unions, and in a landmark move the AMA created its own national negotiating organization, Physicians for Responsible Negotiations (PRN). The goal of this organization is to represent employed physicians and advocate for quality patient care. This 'union' differs from stereotypical unions in that it does not require membership, does not have the ability to strike, use picket lines, or affiliate with other labor groups. Instead, it follows a strict constitution and works with local medical societies to protect the interests of physicians employed by organizations, as opposed to those in private practice.

The Committee of Interns and Residents (CIR) considers itself the voice for interns and residents. It has been joined in a recent legal case against the Boston Medical Center by the AFL-CIO, the American Nurses Association, the California Medical Association, the American Medical Women's Association, and the Medical Society of the State of New York (MSSNY). Arguments submitted to the National Labor Relations Board (NLRB) in Washington, DC, focused on the danger of exploitation of house staff in the increasingly competitive managed care environment. MSSNY concluded, "without any protections [from NLRB] and without any process for dialogue between the hospital and house officers, there may be a greater potential for strife and unrest."

How do IPAs compare to other managed care structures?

IPAs are the least threatening MCOs to physicians because they offer physicians more autonomy than other MCOs. Physicians in IPAs do not have as many practice guidelines imposed on them as do physicians in other structures. In an IPA, the physicians themselves provide health care as they choose, as long as they stay within the reimbursement limitations. For these reasons, IPAs have been highly favored by physicians.

Are IPAs the best option?

Many physicians have joined IPAs because they seemed to be the best option under the managed care system. IPAs have allowed doctors to continue their practices in their own offices and retain a significant amount of autonomy, and have led to only moderate decreases in income. On the other hand, most physicians have little management training and experience. IPAs may not be as successful at cost containment as other structures, and may not have adequate quality assurance processes.

The FTC recently loosened its restraint on physician practices, allowing them to join and collectively compete with HMOs. This policy change led to a more level playing field between HMOs and physician-owned and physician-operated networks. Physicians may increasingly seek to assume more risk and eliminate HMO administration of their practices. The trend may be toward EPOs and PPOs, rather than IPAs, as the favored managed care structures of the future.

Why? Because EPOs and PPOs remove extra levels of administration. The increased efficiency and decreased spending on administrative salaries lower overhead costs. The decreased costs allow them to offer less expensive health-care services to potential employer-customers, thereby increasing their market share of the patient population. The increased market share will then place them in a stronger economic position. However, EPOs and PPOs must be aware that some of the business practices of HMOs grant them a competitive advantage.

What is physician practice management?

Physician practice managements (PPMs) are organizations that contract with physician practices and manage them in exchange for a set fee. These organizations are based on the concept that physicians need management and financial backing to keep their practices viable in a world increasingly dominated by managed care. As such, PPMs are part of an ever-increasing class of management services organizations (MSOs) that offer a range of management and financial services to physician practices.

Although the number of physicians joining PPMs has increased from less than 5,000 in 1995 to more than 15,000 in mid-1997, PPMs face their own challenges. Although increasing numbers of physicians are affiliating with PPMs to be more competitive in the marketplace, local marketplace advantages are very specific, and the ability of a PPM to gain an advantage in one marketplace may not translate into the same advantage in another market.

What are important considerations in joining a PPM?

Before joining a PPM, physicians should consider the performance of other practices acquired by the PPM. The PPM's ability to continue the growth of the practice, sustain stock values, and improve practice efficiencies should be evaluated. Additionally, it is important to inquire about how the PPM funds a practice, and about the involvement of the physicians in this process. A cost-benefit analysis should be included in the analysis to determine if the overall benefits outweigh the often expensive costs in the contract. Finally, it is important to understand the terms that allow a practice to break its contract with a PPM. Although these all seem to be considerable drawbacks to joining a PPM, they have nevertheless been successful in helping practices compete in the managed care marketplace.

Suggested Readings

Lohr KN, Vanselow NA, Detmer DE: The nation's physician workforce: options for balancing supply and requirements. *Institute of Medicine*, 1996.

Mitka M: Working hard for the money. *AMA Medical News* 1996;39(31):1,34.

Seifer SD, Troupin B, Rubenfeld GD: Changes in marketplace demand for physicians: a study of medical journal recruitment advertisements. *JAMA* 1996;276:695-699.

Bindman AB, Grumbach K, Vranizan K, et al: Selection and exclusion of primary care physicians by managed care organizations. *JAMA* 1998;279:675-679.

Kuttner R: Must good HMOs go bad? First of two parts: the commercialization of prepaid group health care. *N Engl J Med* 1998;338:1558-1563.

Antitrust relief. *AMA Medical News* 1996;39(36):17.

Franklin H: CIR wins wide backing as labor board hears BMC case. *Committee of Interns and Residents News* 1998;27(1):9.

New antitrust policy offers big gains for doctor networks. *AMA Medical News* 1996;39(35):1,34-35.

Reardon T: Doctors, unions often not a good match. *AMA Medical News*, March 23/30, 1998.

Drake DF: Managed care. A product of market dynamics. *JAMA* 1997;277:560-563.

Kuttner R: Physician-operated networks and the new antitrust guidelines. *N Engl J Med* 1997;336:386-391.

Robinson JC: Consolidation of medical groups into physician practice management organizations. *JAMA* 1998;279:144-149.

Tokarski C: Running the obstacle course. *AMA Medical News*, April 13, 1998.

Chapter 9

Medicare and Medicaid

The sources of health-care funding in the United States include private insurance companies, the government, and employers' and patients' out-of-pocket payments. Government funding accounts for the bulk of health-care expenditures; expenditures amounted to more than 45% of health-care costs ($411.7 billion) in 1996. Out-of-pocket expenditures amounted to 19% of personal health-care expenditures ($171.8 billion) and insurance companies paid 32% of health-care costs ($292.4 billion). Today an even higher fraction of expenditures are from government and insurance sources, with less expenditures from out-of-pocket sources. Because the government spends the most money on health care, cutbacks in government spending have been a common theme in much of the legislation to curb health-care costs (Figure 1).

What is Medicare?

Title XVIII of the Social Security Act, or Medicare, as it is more commonly known, was initiated July 1, 1966, to provide medical care for the senior citizen population (those over 65) who were covered by Social Security. Medicare eligibility is not based on need: the only criterion is age. In 1972, amendments to Medi-

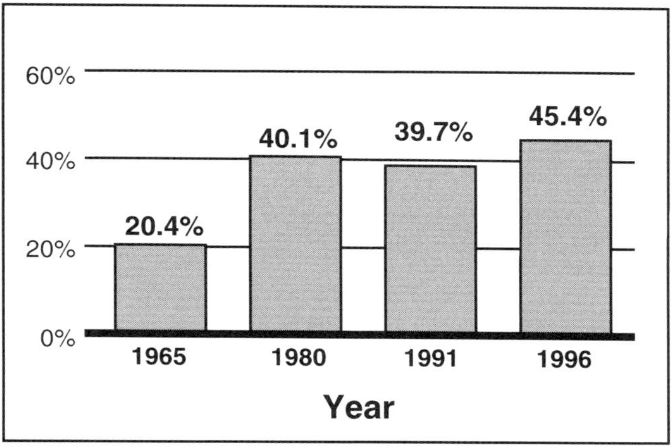

Figure 1: Health care costs paid by public sector.

care extended coverage to people 65 or older who are not covered by the Social Security system, but who are willing to pay small premiums. Medicare benefits were further extended to individuals with certain disabilities (qualifying under the disabilities clause of the Social Security Act), and to people suffering from chronic kidney disease requiring hemodialysis. Hemodialysis was included as a specific part of Medicare because of its lack of availability at the time, a decision that set precedents for health-care policy today (Table 1).

Most managed care organizations (MCOs) argue that funds for hemodialysis are being used inappropriately. MCOs maintain that the $12 billion for treating end-stage renal disease can be decreased with new ways of providing hemodialysis at home.

What is the difference between Part A and Part B of Medicare?

Part A of Medicare is financed by payroll taxes collected under Social Security. It covers hospital care, ex-

Table 1: The Impact of Hemodialysis

- Hemodialysis ushered in capitated programs
- Diagnosis-related groups (DRGs) started with hemodialysis
- Hemodialysis ushered in home care
- Hemodialysis was the government's first significant experience with disease-specific, universal coverage
- Hemodialysis has grown into a $12 billion market

tended care in a facility, and patient home care. The entire cost of Part A is paid by the Medicare Trust Fund, which is a separate government account funded by additions to each worker's Social Security tax. Part B is a voluntary supplemental program that pays for physician's services and other medical expenses. It is funded by taxes and contributions paid by the patient (Table 2).

Simply put, Part A pays the hospitals, and Part B pays the physicians. An important part of Medicare is that neither Part A nor Part B provides comprehensive care. Take the following example of a hypothetical extended stay at a hospital:

Day 1:	Patient pays deductible for first day care (which was set in 1987 at $520)
Days 2-60:	Patient pays 25% of the cost, Medicare pays the rest
Days 91-150:	Patient pays 50% of cost, Medicare pays the rest
Days beyond 150:	Medicare pays nothing

Table 2: Financing of Medicare

	Part A	Part B
What is covered?	Hospital care, extended care	Physician's services, other medical expenses home care
Who pays for it?	Payroll taxes (Social Security)	Taxes and contributions paid by the patient

While this simplifies how Medicare reimburses patients, it does illustrate one of the major problems with Medicare: it provides no serious protection against catastrophic illnesses. A catastrophic illness is one that requires an extended stay at a hospital, a situation that could bankrupt most middle-income families. This has led to the growth of Medigap insurance to cover these deficiencies in Medicare. Medigap is a supplemental insurance offered by various private companies at an additional cost to the patient.

What is Medicaid?

Both Medicaid and Medicare are government programs created by the Johnson administration in the late 1960s. However, they serve different populations, and funds are managed differently. Medicaid was designed to provide medical care to the poor, blind, and disabled. Medicaid also covers families with dependent children if one parent is 'absent, unemployed, or unable to work.' This care is financed equally by both federal and state sources, and is administered by the individual states, unlike Medicare. Each state determines the eligibility of Medicaid applicants. People already receiving financial aid from the state often are eligible for Medicaid. Table 3 outlines Medicaid benefits.

Table 3: Medicaid Coverage

- Inpatient and outpatient care
- Laboratory and x-ray services
- Physician services
- Nursing facility and home health services
- Family planning
- Preventive medicine services

How has managed care affected Medicare and Medicaid?

Many states have encouraged Medicare and Medicaid enrollees to join private managed care programs. This would transfer responsibility for their health care from the state to the MCO. The current reimbursement system allows Medicare to pay an MCO 95% of what Medicare would have spent on the average enrollee, therefore saving 5% of these funds. The MCO may then lower costs by controlling the use of resources, just as the MCO would for any other enrollee. However, such a relationship may be corrupted by the MCO, which could restrict use of resources or attempt to control patient enrollment, raising issues of quality maintenance.

Medicaid is also shifting toward becoming integrated with MCOs in many states, and is faced with many of the same hurdles. In New York, for example, the transition of Medicaid to managed care has flooded the MCOs with the states' 2.8 million participants, resulting in complaints of decreased level of care.

How are physicians reimbursed under Medicare?

Medicare pays physicians using the fee-for-service system. Medicare, when it was first introduced by President Lyndon B. Johnson in 1966, included a set fee schedule to compensate physicians. At the time, physicians generally opposed Medicare, fearing that the government would set reimbursements at lower rates, thereby decreasing their income. Eventually, a system was created in which physicians could bill the government according to the "usual and customary prevailing fee," defined as less than the 75th percentile of fees charged by all physicians in a community.

In 1992, the Omnibus Budget Reconciliation Act of 1989 (OBRA) changed physician compensation through Medicare. The new resource-based-relative-value scale (RBRVS) assigned a *relative value* based on the required time, skill, and intensity to perform a service. This system contrasted with the earlier fee-for-service system, which favored procedures over nonprocedure services. The relative values are adjusted according to geographic variations and multiplied by a national conversion factor to determine the actual dollar amount. For example, a simple examination or procedure performed by a generalist and a specialist would be reimbursed similarly because the time, skill, and intensity involved is the same; specialists would not be reimbursed more because of their specialty. By limiting what physicians could charge and by reimbursing less for costly specialist procedures than for generalist procedures, Congress hoped that the RBRVS would limit the growth of health-care expenditures. However, data have shown that the RBRVS system has not decreased physician compensation as much as anticipated. Many physicians order additional procedures to increase the number of reimbursements. For example, a patient with cystic fibrosis may also have chronic obstructive pulmonary disease (COPD) included in the diagnosis to indicate additional examinations or procedures.

Unlike Medicare, Medicaid reimbursement to physicians is controlled by the states, which provide 50% of the funding. Therefore, the physician should inquire

Table 4: Causes of Medicare and Medicaid overspending

- Coverage of new services
- Coverage of costlier services
- Increased lifespan/population
- Increased health-care demands by an aging population

into the reimbursement method used by Medicaid in his or her state.

How have Medicare and Medicaid increased health-care expenditures?

Health-care expenditures have skyrocketed over the last 20 years, not just in governmental programs. The 20.4% of personal health-care expenditures paid by the public sector in 1965 increased to 40% in 1980, and to 45.4% in 1996 (Figure 1). Medicare and Medicaid payments have exceeded their projected expenditures since their creation. Severe overspending has been caused by new services added to benefit packages, increased life span of beneficiaries, aging baby boomers demanding more health care, and the coverage of costlier procedures such as dialysis and transplants (Table 4).

In summary, the dramatic rise in federal expenditures can be linked to the creation of Medicare and Medicaid in 1966, which assigned the government the role of third-party payer (Figure 2). This favors a system of overutilization. Physicians who performed more services made more money, while patients were unaware of health-care costs. Because the government paid the bills, physicians provided maximal care to patients, regardless of cost. Additionally, highly techni-

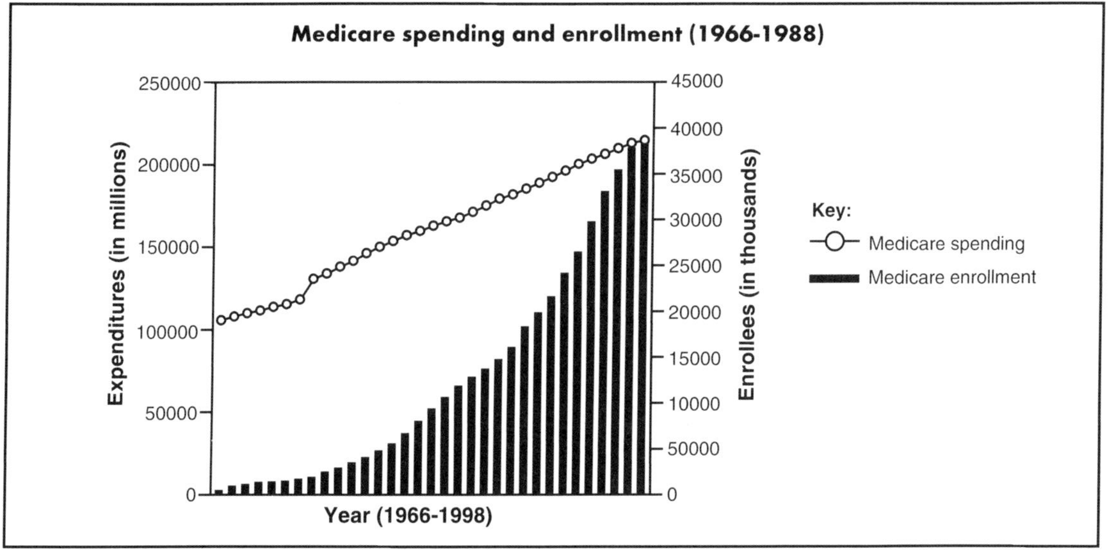

Figure 2: Both the number of enrollees and the amount of spending has increased over the life of Medicare (Presented from data from the Health Care Financing Administration: financial information not corrected for annual inflation).

cal services reimbursed by Medicare (eg, magnetic resonance imaging) experienced an explosive rate of growth in the 1970s and 1980s. The growth and unrestricted use of medical technology such as hemodialysis has further increased health-care expenditures.

Will Medicare and Medicaid funding be cut?

Reductions in Medicare spending are expected in the near future, in response to projections that the Medicare trust fund will be depleted early in the 21st century. When negotiations over the federal balanced-budget bill ended in 1996, the Clinton administration agreed to a $124 billion cut in Medicare spending over a 7-year period.

What are the effects of Medicare cuts on hospitals?

Over the next 5 years, $116 billion will be cut out of Medicare. Under the Balanced Budget Act of 1997, hospitals would receive almost $40 billion less in Medicare payments. This also translates to a $16 billion loss for the home health-care industry, and a $10 billion loss for nursing homes. This could force many community hospitals, nursing homes, and home health-care providers to find other ways to remain solvent. A popular trend today is for these facilities to associate with larger MCOs to survive. Cuts in Medicare will accelerate the mergers and consolidations of community hospitals with larger hospital chains.

With the introduction of RBRVS to Medicare, patients have shorter hospital stays. For example, when an elderly patient breaks a hip, the typical hospital stay is 7 days. A decade ago, the minimum stay was 10 days. While RBRVS was meant to cap Medicare spending, in some respects it has done just the opposite. Patients were often sent home before they were fully recovered. Many of these patients transferred to nursing homes where their care was covered by Medicare, often at more than $400 a day. In short,

Medicare became a boon to home health-care providers and nursing homes that made large profits off of Medicare reimbursements.

What will be the effects of Medicare cuts on physicians?

Physicians whose incomes are primarily based on Medicare will have their incomes drastically endangered. Geriatrics, the specialty most obviously affected by changes in Medicare, is no different. The Balanced Budget Act will allow patients to choose between fee-for-service, managed care, or medical savings accounts. It will also increase reimbursements to office-based primary care physicians and for preventative services. Such changes prompted Ettinger to state that despite decreased reimbursements, there will be opportunities for physicians to continue to control the care of their patients. Nonetheless, many physicians foresee future difficulties in being reimbursed.

Changes in Medicare are not limited to reimbursements. New evaluation and management (E&M) guidelines proposed by the Health Care Financing Administration (HCFA) require physicians to carefully document health care services rendered for reimbursment. Many physicians see the new E&M guidelines as excessively cumbersome and a hindrance to their practice. The ideal practice is set up with several sources of income, ie, not solely dependent on Medicare.

Suggested Readings

Home is where the hemo is. *AMA Medical News*, October 7, 1996.

Wilson N: *Health Services in the United States*, 1982.

Kovner AR: *Jonas's Healthcare Delivery in the United States*, 5th ed. New York, Springer, 1995.

Pear R: Bill would sever Medicaid benefits from welfare aid. *N Y Times*, December 12, 1995.

Fisher I, Fein EB: Forced marriage of Medicaid and managed care hits snags. *N Y Times*, August 28, 1995.

Newhouse et al: *Rand Corporation's Health Insurance Experiment, 1981*. Phelps, Health Economics.

The New York Health Care Community: 1997 and Beyond. Greater New York Hospital Association, September 1996.

Ettinger WH: The Balanced Budget Act of 1997: Implications for the practice of geriatric medicine *J Am Geriatr Soc* 1998;46:530-533.

Chapter **10**

Afterword

Throughout this book, we have attempted to clearly describe various managed care concepts. This material should help medical students, physicians, and other health professionals understand both the present health-care environment and the changes that may come.

Several other issues are important, however. First, local and regional differences exist among the various managed care systems. Managed care takes different meanings for different people in different places. Knowing managed care basics is not enough. Physicians must also be aware of how managed care is applied in the local environment.

Second, trends in the health-care marketplace tend to be cyclical. Although the recent health-care trend involves a shift away from specialist care, this trend is not new. Before the popularity of specialist care, there was indeed a preference for and prevalence of primary care physicians. Such cyclical trends have existed for many years, and will most likely continue. While it is prudent to be informed of the health-care market and current managed care preferences, the ultimate decision to enter a primary care or specialty field, or the decision about which managed care system is best, should be influenced by factors other than the health-care cycle. Personality, lifestyle preference, and technical ability should play significant roles in the career decisions of new and young physicians.

Finally, managed care is a dynamic concept; changes are constant. Although the present focus may be on low cost, many MCOs are repositioning toward providing quality health care. Considering the rapid pace of such changes, we encourage readers to stay informed about the development of managed care. Periodicals and newsletters from professional organizations (such as the American Medical Association, American Medical Students Association, and Association of American Medical Colleges) can help physicians stay abreast of proposed legislation and local and national changes. As physicians, we cannot afford to sit still while the health-care market develops around us. We must stay informed and involved.

Chapter **11**

Glossary

Capitation - A fixed amount of money paid to a provider for health-care services. This amount is calculated using cost of visit and average number of visits. For example, a third-party payer may pay: $120/visit × average of 3 visits per member divided by 12 months/year = $30 per member per month for all care for that member.

Case management - The process by which all health-related matters of a case are managed by a physician or other health professional. Case managers coordinate components of health care, such as appropriate referral to consultants, specialists, hospitals, and other providers. Case management is intended to ensure continuity of services and to decrease misuse of facilities and resources, particularly in chronic or more severe cases.

Claims review - The method by which an enrollee's health-care service claims are reviewed before reimbursement. The purpose is to validate the medical necessity of the provided services to be sure the cost and use of the services are not excessive.

Closed panel - Physicians who only serve the managed care organization (MCO) deliver medical services in an MCO-owned health center or satellite clinic. This term usually refers to a group or staff model HMO.

Co-payment (co-pay) - The fixed amount of money that a member pays out of his or her own pocket every time services are rendered. For example, a patient may be required to pay $10 for every visit to a doctor and the third-party payer pays the balance of the fee.

Diagnosis Related Groups (DRGs) - A cost-control mechanism in which reimbursement for a given patient is determined before the delivery of any health care based on diagnosis. For example, a patient presenting with a specific disease will be covered for predetermined amount based on the projected cost to treat that disease.

Fee-for-service - The traditional payment method whereby patients pay doctors, hospitals, and other providers for services rendered and then bill private insurers or the government.

Formulary - A list of drugs to which physicians are restricted. A physician may use a nonformulary medication if there is a valid medical reason. Physicians are generally not compensated for prescribing drugs not in the formulary.

Gag rules (clauses) - Limits imposed on practitioners (not only doctors, but also nurses, physician substitutes, etc) by the MCO regarding the practitioners' discussion with patients' various treatment options, usually those either more costly, or those not covered by the plan.

Gatekeeper - A clinician (usually a primary care physician) whose role it is to control the *gate* to further specialist care, as well as manage all the care delivered to an enrollee.

Group Model - An HMO that contracts with a medical group for the provision of health-care services to members of the HMO. A form of closed panel health plan.

Health Maintenance Organization (HMO) -
Old definition: - An organization, either nonprofit or for-profit, that accepts responsibility for providing and delivering a predetermined set of comprehensive health maintenance and treatment services to a voluntarily enrolled population for a prenegotiated, capitated amount.
Recent definition: - Old definition plus: the placement of providers at risk for medical expenses. Simply put, physicians are financially responsible for keeping costs down.

Indemnity - A form of health insurance in which insurers pay for services (fee-for-service) provided by physicians. In the indemnity system, few rules restrict which, when, or how often a specialist is seen or procedures are performed.

Independent Practice Association (IPA) - An organization consisting of independent physicians that obtains contracts with managed care plans. The organization is paid at a capitated rate as reimbursement for health-care services delivered to the members of the managed care plans.

Managed Care Organization (MCO) - A generic term applied to various managed care plan models.

Member - An individual (enrollee) enrolled for health services or benefits (see Subscriber).

Mixed model - A managed care plan that combines two or more types of systems, eg, generally used to describe an HMO that has features of both an open and closed panel.

National Committee for Quality Assurance (NCQA) - A nonprofit organization that reviews the accreditation of managed care organizations. The reviews are based on quality.

Network model - A managed care plan that contracts with more than one group of physicians for delivery of comprehensive health care to their members.

Open panel - A managed care plan that allows members to seek care from physicians who are not contracted with the plan. Members are then responsible for a greater portion of the bill. Examples of open panel plans are the IPA, PPO, or POS.

Participating provider - May apply to either professional or institutional providers who have contracted with a managed care plan.

Primary Care Physician (PCP) - Refers to the fields of internal medicine, pediatrics, and family medicine/general practice; occasionally to obstetrics/gynecology.

Physician Hospital Organization (PHO) - Affiliations of hospitals and physicians (often the attending medical staff), usually involving direct contracts and risk sharing, in order to compete with managed care plans.

Per Member Per Month (PMPM) - An amount in reference to each enrolled member each month.

Per Member Per Year (PMPY) - Same concept as PMPM, but per year.

Physician group - Two or more physicians who share resources and distribute profits among themselves.

Point of Service (POS) - A plan in which members choose how and when they receive needed services. There is generally an out-of-pocket cost to members who opt for POS and who use nonplan providers. For example, a patient may go to a nonplan provider for an additional fee.

Pre-certification - The process of obtaining authorization from the managed care plan for a given service before obtaining that service. Failure to contact your plan in advance generally results in a financial penalty to the member, often with denial of coverage.

Risk sharing - Utilization control mechanism in which the physician is included in the chance or possibility of loss from substantial medical charges.

Staff model - An early version of HMO in which physicians are employed directly by the HMO to provide services in an HMO-owned facility; a form of closed panel HMO.

Subscriber - The person in whose name an individual or family contract is issued.

Third party - Individual or company that contracts with employers who want to self-insure the health of their employees. They develop and coordinate self-insurance programs, process and pay the claims.

Utilization Review (UR) - Also known as utilization management or utilization control. UR is a systematic means for reviewing and controlling patients' use of medical services as well as the appropriateness and quality of that care.

Withholds - Used by MCOs to include physicians in risk sharing. The MCO sets aside a certain amount of money from the physicians' salaries each month. If the physicians save money by limiting treatments and tests, the leftover money at the end of the month is divided among the plan's physicians. An issue here is that money becomes an incentive to limit health care.

Index

A

B

C

K

L

M

N